Food
For
Ageless Look

Anti-aging food list for 40's and beyond

By Beatrice .K. MacBrown

Copyright

Disclaimer

This book is projected to be a general guide to raise consciousness and aid people in making knowledgeable decisions in their circumstances. This book's content is not expected to be a replacement for professional medical advice, diagnosis, or treatment.

The author takes no responsibility for any damage or injury, be it personal or monetary, due to the use or abuse of the information in this book. If you have any doubts or worries after reading this book, do well to speak to a qualified person before further actions.

Table of contents

Chapter One

Anti-aging food

Aging is a process that comes naturally, you can't stop aging, and no man can reverse it, but you can delay it early onset by staying healthy. To have good health in your senior years, you must eat right.

Feeling your best and staying healthy, you need to feed yourself with proper nutrition for it to function properly. Good maintenance on your body is important at any age and oh don't forget that your body is a machine, a well-oiled machine.

As the year passes, our bodies begin to change in all areas ranging from how we look to how our bodies accept things.

For examples eating food you once desire become a problem simply because you have lost interest in eating, what about chewing, automatically that also becomes a nightmare. All these happened and keep us from eating well because our body is undergoing an inevitable change.

We can slow the rate of this transformation called aging by our food intake.

If we make it a habit to consume foods loaded with healthy fats, antioxidants, water, and essential nutrients, our bodies will thank us for that by showing healthy and glowing skins.

Healthy Diet

The human body needs essentials nutrients to perform simple functions, if the body is not provided with enough of the required nutrients, aging will set in pretty fast.

Choose the right foods and give up the wrong ones, and the whole part of your body will be nourished for years to come.

Healthy diets are eating lots of fruits and vegetables, whole grains, healthy protein, low-fat dairy and healthy fats. The above food lists are beneficial for an older adult who desire to eat healthier.

Water though not food, but should be included as a healthy diet. The urge to drink water reduces as we get older, don't give in to that, try drinking as much water as possible to revitalize your cells.

What you eat tell who you are, your diet has a significant effect on your health. Do you want to look younger than ever as you age gracefully?

If the answer is yes, you need discipline to stick like glue to the following listed habits:

- o Healthy diets
- o Regular exercise
- o Nightly sleep of at least seven hours
- o Detailed skin care regimen

Regular consumption of anti-aging food has a lot of health benefit, especially for the 40s and beyond. The following are a few benefits of eating anti-aging food.

The hair will be healthy

Nails become stronger

Trim and Slim figure.

Reduction in the risk of diabetes and heart disease

Better circulation of blood

Lower blood pressure

Youthful and glowing skin

Looking good and healthy is only a step away, include all the anti-aging food on your diet, and you will not depend on anti-aging treatment and cream to look younger ever again.

We are talking about what you eat.

Chapter Two

Seeds and Nuts

- Sesame seeds

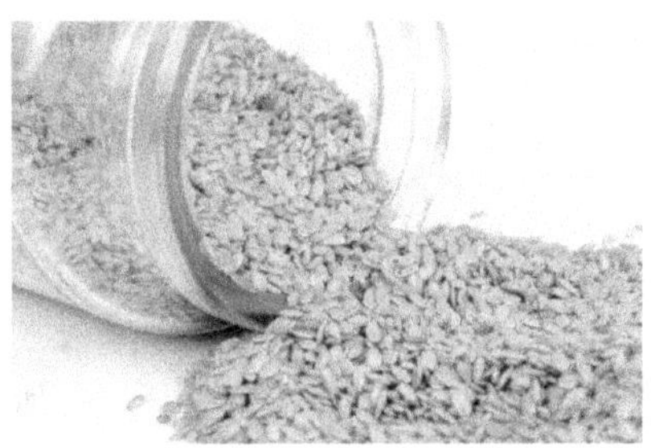

Sesame seeds are delicious and contain a type of lignin called sesamin.

Sesamin is a phytoestrogen that has anti-aging effects on the body. Sesame is rich in calcium, magnesium, iron, phosphorous and fiber. Adding sesame in your diet will help to maintain healthy and strong bone. Chewing it raw every morning gives a glowing skin.

- **Nuts**

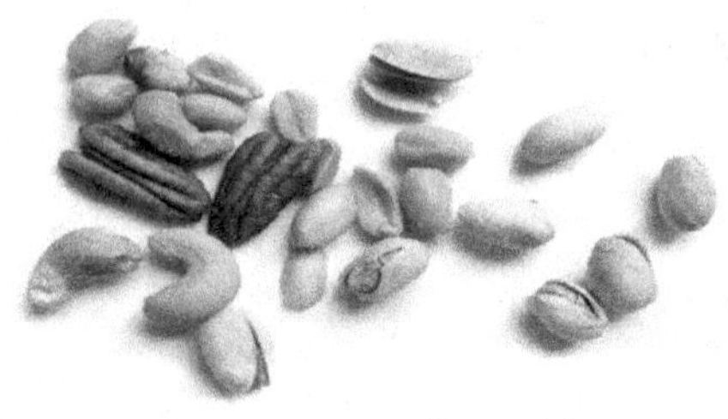

Consuming one or two handfuls of mixed nuts like almonds, cashews, pistachios, pecans, and any other nuts everyday help to delay signs of aging. These nuts are packed with essential vitamins such as protein, phytosterols, and cholesterol-reducing fiber.

- **Walnut**

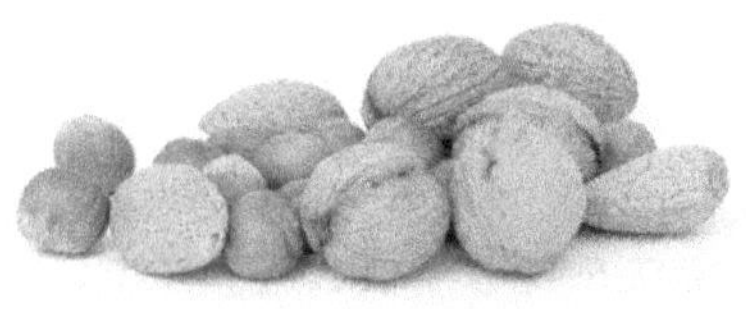

Walnut is high in antioxidant and other nutrients. It contains gamma-tocopherols, an anti-inflammatory compound that reduces the inflammation level on the body, thereby decreasing the aging effect on the body. The presence of anti-oxidants in walnuts helps prevent damage caused by the sun and eliminate toxin that cause early aging. Regular intake of walnut reverses age-linked motor and cognitive degeneration giving you that youthful and fresh skin.

- Beans and lentils

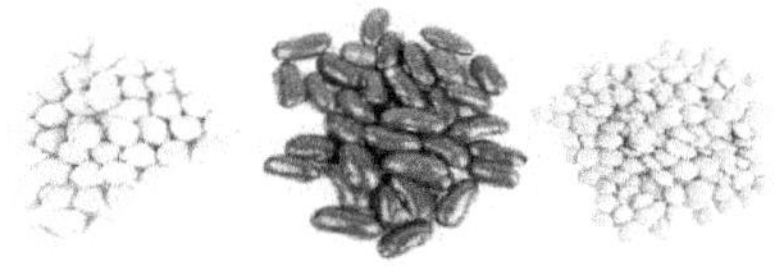

Beans and lentils are loads with essential amino acid (plant-based) that take care of all protein requirements, this amino acid fuel, and boost body energy. A lentil contains a lot of vitamin B9, which can prevent balding and gray hairs. Increase your beans and lentil intake as you grow older because they are enriched with phytochemicals and disease-fighting fiber.

- Oatmeal

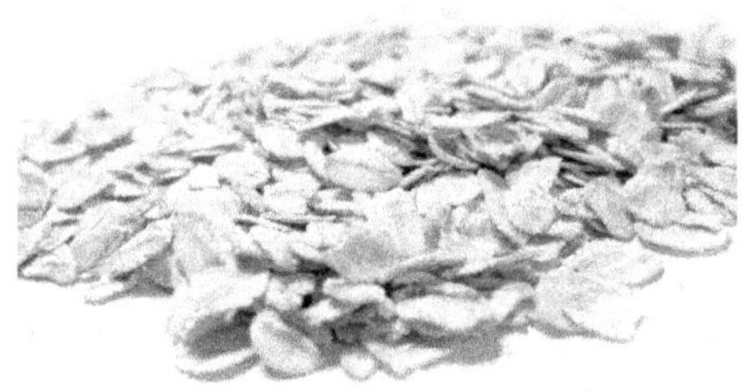

Oatmeal is packed with zinc and iron, which boosts hair and nail growth. Oatmeal contains a strong antioxidant compound known as avenanthramide that helps in slowing down the rate of aging. Oatmeal is also rich in carbohydrates and it makes the body feel young, and hearty. Eat a bowl of oatmeal for breakfast and get the sensational anti-aging feeling.

- Pomegranate seeds

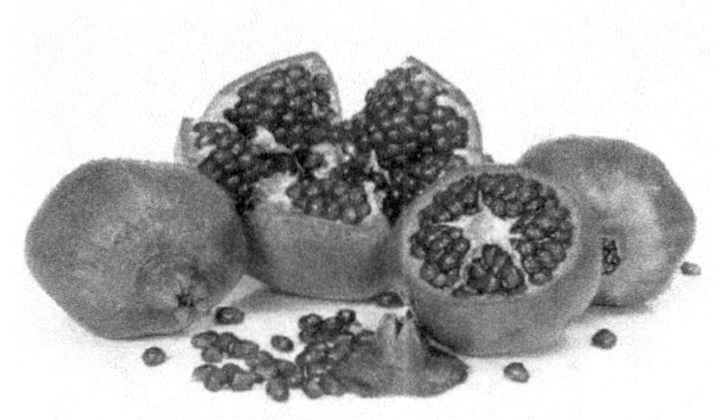

Pomegranate is enriched with important compounds like Vitamins C, D, E and K, magnesium, selenium and protein. All these compound work together to increase the body's ability to preserve collagen and also fight damage from free radicals. Regular consumption of pomegranate has an anti-aging effect on the body.

Add the tasty and crunchy fruit to your meal, and your skin will look younger in years to come.

- Pumpkin Seed

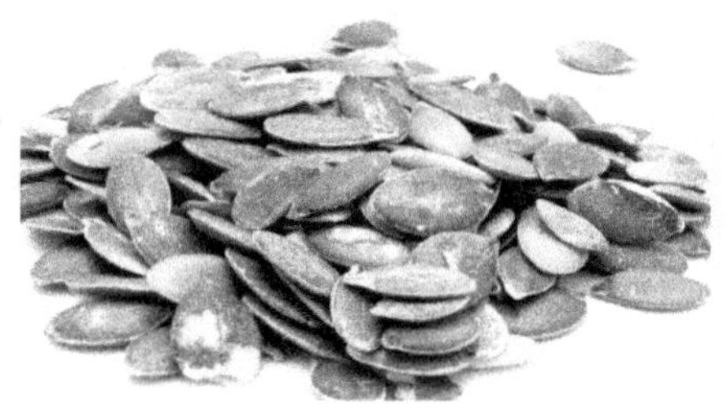

Pumpkin seed is a great seed with many nutritional values. They are high in monounsaturated fats and amino acids, which fight depression, sleep disorder and improve mood.

Chapter Three

Fruits

- Blueberries

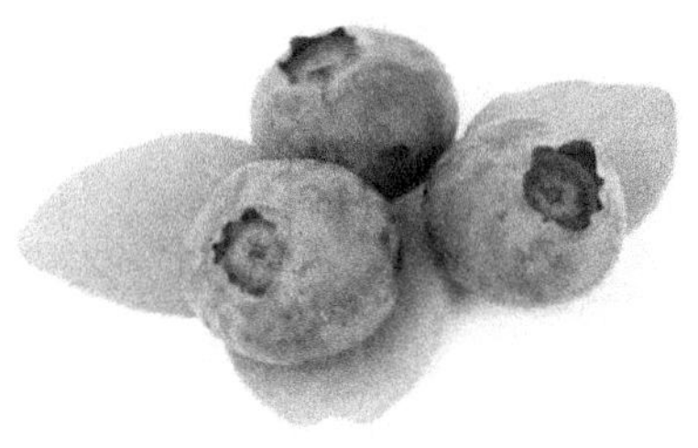

Blueberries are endowed with antioxidants properties more than any other berries or fruits. The antioxidant properties protect the skin against free radicals from exposure to sun, stress, and pollution. The blueberries are rich in phytochemical whose function is to limit the development of neurodegenerative diseases of aging. The presence of vitamin C in blueberries helps to prevent wrinkles.

- **Pineapple**

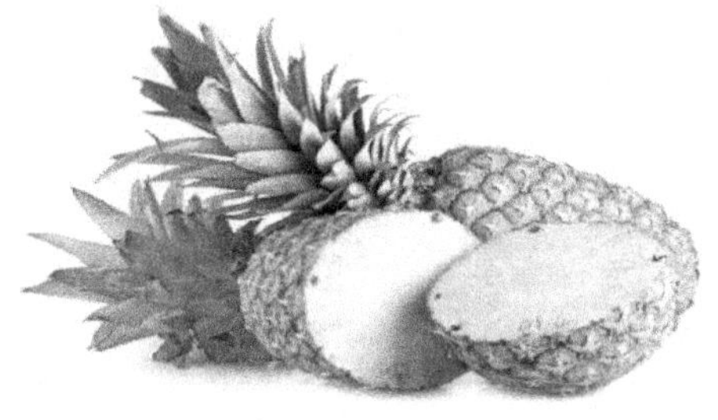

Pineapple is one of the best anti-aging foods readily available. It is rich in manganese minerals and other vital nutrients such as Vitamin B, Vitamin C, fiber, testosterone, and phosphorous. The Prolidase enzymes in pineapple make available the amino acid proline, which forms collagen in the skin. Collagen gives skin strength and elasticity.

- **Lemon and lime water**

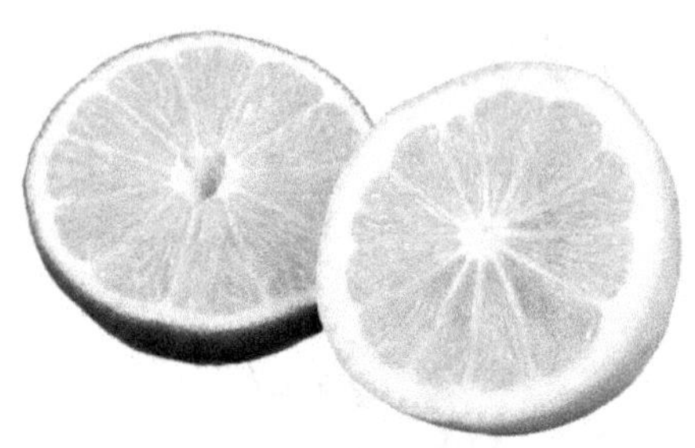

Lemon and lime are vitamin C rich citrus that plays an essential role in maintaining ideal genetic health.

Vitamin C is an essential antioxidant that defends the skin from the harmful effects of free radicals. People who consume much of lemon-lime water keep their skin looking brighter, smoother, and younger and have fewer wrinkles. Regular consumption of lemon-lime water improves the presence of dull skin and wrinkles in middle-aged women. It also decreases the aging process.

- Orange

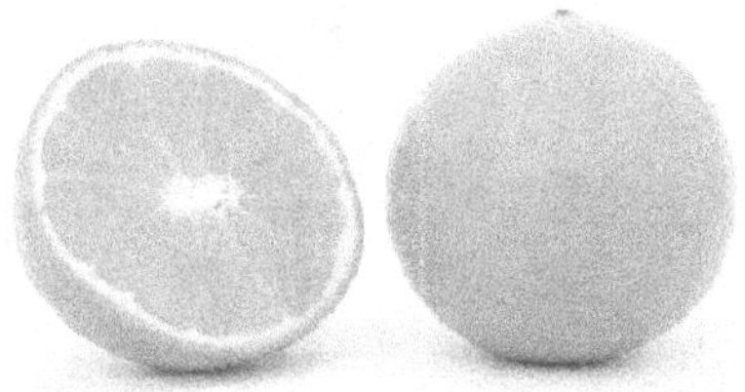

Orange is an anti-aging fruit. Regular intake of oranges naturally boosts the body's collagen production. The collagen present in oranges when consumed makes the skin more supple, dewy, and younger-looking. The high content of vitamin C in orange helps boost the immune system and gives the body relief from any symptom of a cold.

- Watermelon

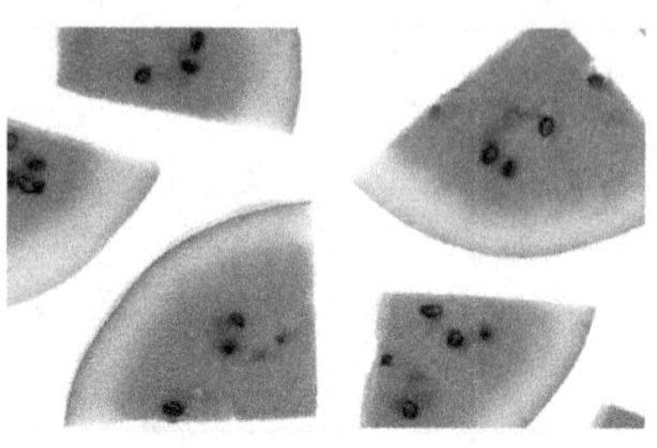

Watermelon boosts your intake of water greatly during hot and humid days. It does not stop at that; it also protects the skin from premature aging, hydrated, and plump. Watermelon is enriched with lycopene, which function is to protect the skin from ultraviolet rays that age and damage the skin. Watermelon has a high content of vitamins C, E, and K, calcium, selenium, manganese, protein, potassium, and carbohydrates.

- **Olives**

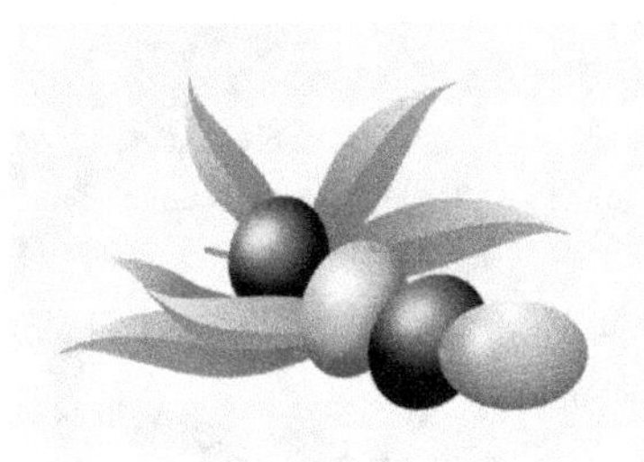

Olives are an excellent source of polyphenols and phytonutrients that help protect DNA and give more energy and younger feeling. These beneficial nutrients can only be found in fresh olives, not canned ones. Canned olives are strip off their vital nutrient during the pitting process. Regular consumption of a small quantity of olive helps to prevent wrinkles and blemishes caused by old age.

- **Avocado**

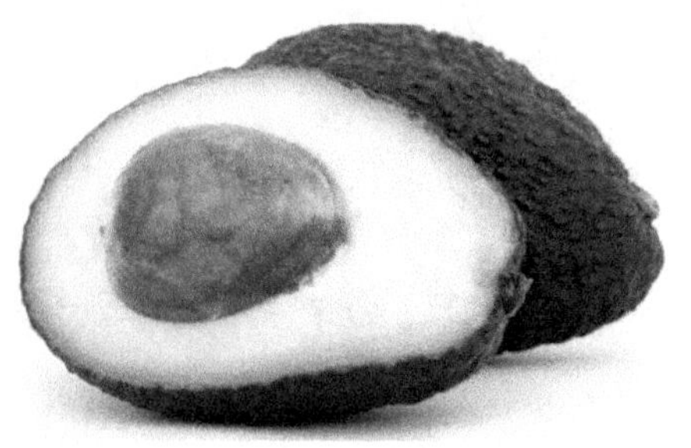

Avocado is rich in vitamins A, C, E, and K, potassium and antioxidants that combat the effect of aging. The fatty acids present in avocado help fight inflammation to boost the immune system, brain and the overall body. Add avocado in your meal regularly to give you that youthful feeling and look.

You can use it for toast, salad or pudding.

- **Papaya**

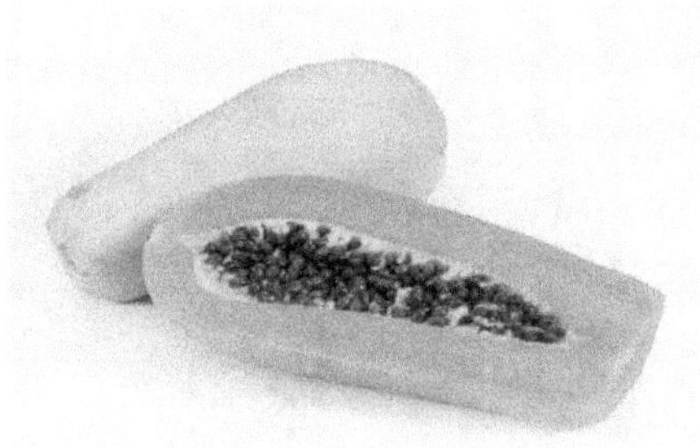

Papaya is enriched with an enzyme called Papain which helps the body in shedding dead skin cells. The enzyme is usually seen in most exfoliating products. Papaya is enriched with vital vitamins and minerals that delay the sign of aging in the skin. The beneficial nutrients in papaya are vitamins A, B, C, K and E, potassium, calcium, magnesium and phosphorus.

- **Figs**

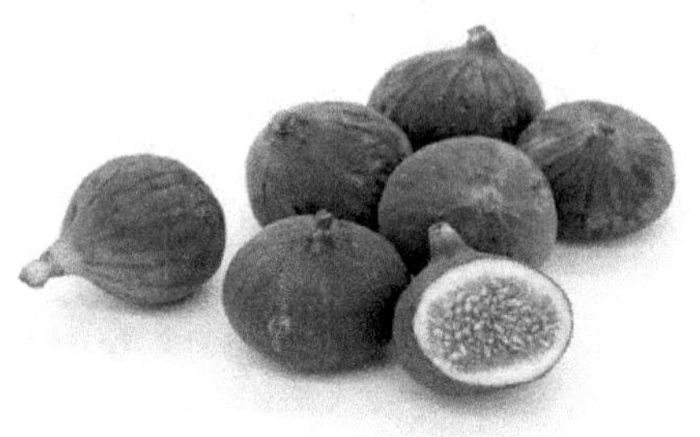

Fig fruits are packed with polyphenols and flavonoids compounds, which help to take away free radicals from the cells of the skin. The anti-oxidants property present in figs helps in slowing down the effect of aging in the body. Add fig to your meal regularly to keep your skin and system healthy.

- **Strawberries**

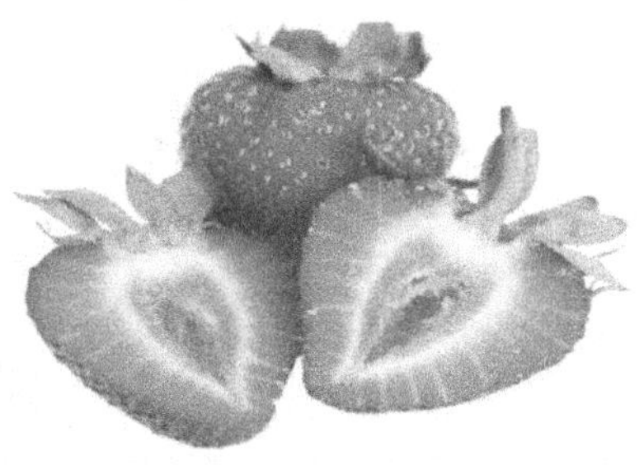

Strawberry has a great taste and very high in essential micronutrients like vitamin C and anthocyanin. They have antioxidant and anti-inflammatory properties that boost cellular metabolism and revive dead cell by reducing oxidative stress and significantly reducing the effect of aging.

Regular addition of this yummy fruit in your diet makes all the difference.

- Grapefruit

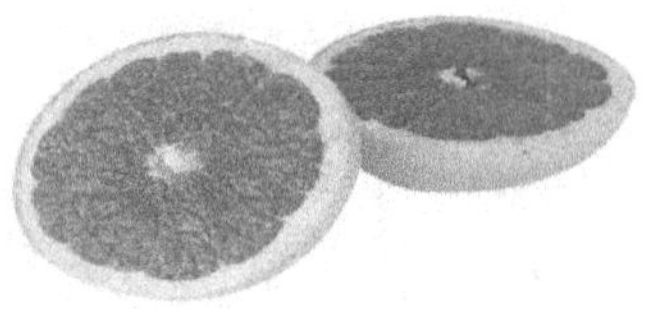

Grapefruit contains a high amount of vitamin C and spermidine. These nutrients are known to reduce effect of the aging in human immune cells. Next time you come across grapefruit, stop by and pick one .Always consult your doctor before taking grapefruit.

- Guavas

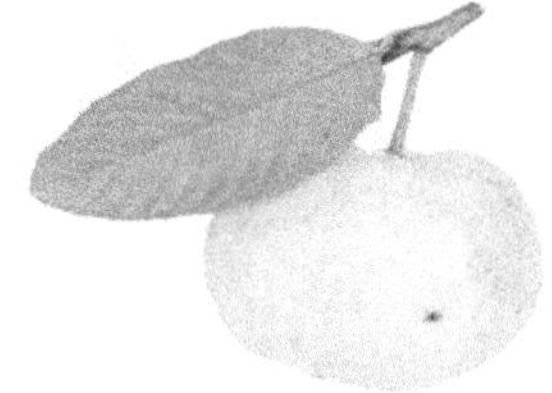

Guava is another great fruit that is rich in Vitamins C, potassium, and antioxidants. Regular consumption of guava reduces the effect of aging significantly.

Chapter Four

Vegetables

- **Broccoli**

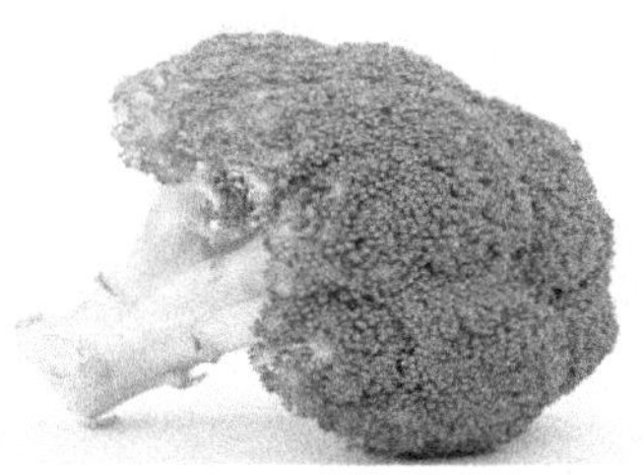

Broccoli contains lutein, which is a plant pigment found in vegetables. The high content of antioxidant in broccoli helps in fighting off aging signs. Regular consumption of broccoli gives a better mental cognition and job performance that needs intelligence.

- **Carrots**

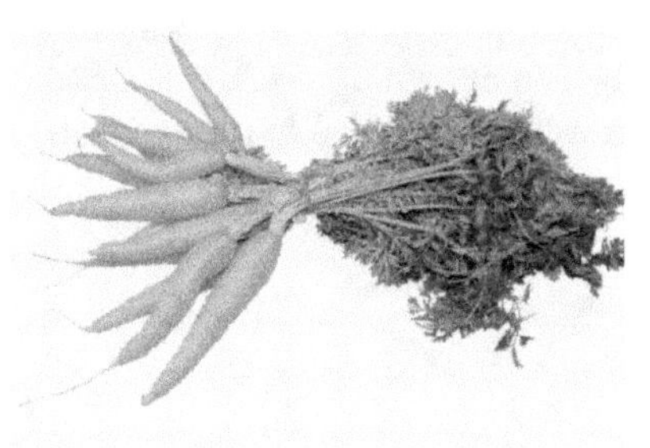

Carrots are crunchy and tasty vegetables and are a great source of beta-carotene, anti-oxidants, and potassium. Carrots have abundant of vitamin A which regenerates the skin cells and restores its elasticity (collagen). It is a healthy snack that has impressive cancer-fighting properties.

Add carrots to your meal for healthy and glowing skin.

- Edamame

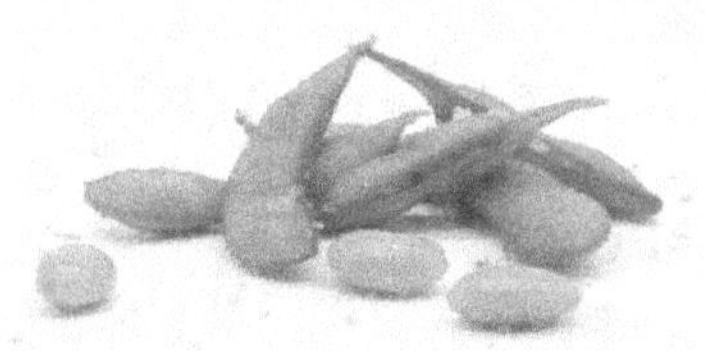

Edamame is an unprocessed soy food that
wrinkles and skin fine lines when
consumed for at least three consecutive
months. It can take you back to the days
when you have wrinkles free face and soft
skin. Edamame is also high in maintaining
healthy bones and improving the
cardiovascular system. It helps women
who have reached their menopause by
providing phytoestrogen compounds,
which increases their estrogen level,
thereby preventing loss of bones and risk
of heart disease.

- Mushrooms

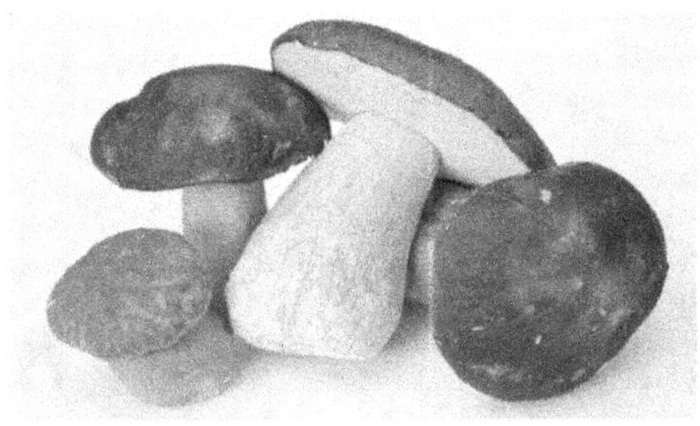

Mushrooms are one of the anti-aging foods that naturally contain vitamin D. Presence of vitamin D in the body help in proper absorption of calcium, which will lead to stronger bones and spine. Most mushrooms contain vital essential vitamins, but shiitake mushrooms are a great source of copper. Copper is anti-aging vitamins that help delay or partly lessen the greying hair process. Regular snacking on shiitake mushroom may put to a hold the inevitable graying process.

- Cooked tomatoes

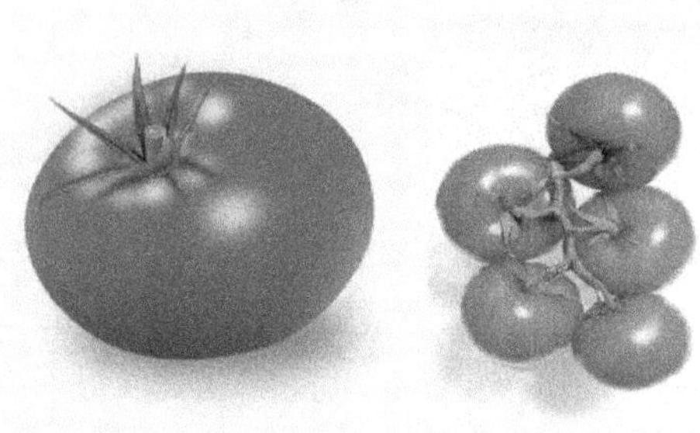

Tomatoes contain more anti-aging properties when they are cooked. Cooked tomatoes are loaded with lycopene, a non-provitamin A carotenoid that protects the skin from UV rays' damage. Raw tomatoes also provide the body with lycopene, but the cooking process makes it less difficult to be absorbed in the body system. The outer part of the tomato has an anti-inflammatory result on the skin, and the flavonoids content in the fruit slows down aging.

- **Watercress**

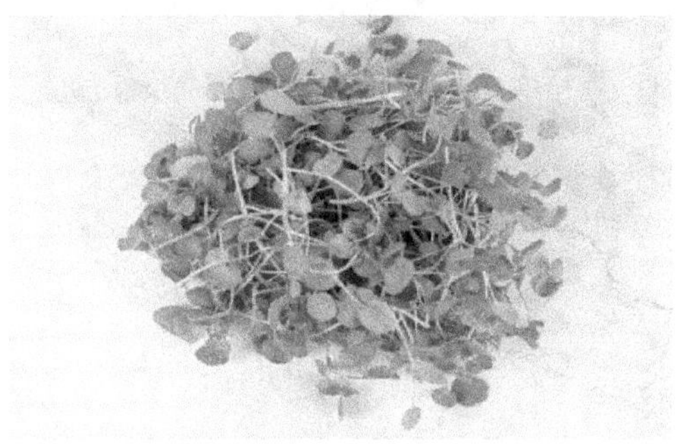

Watercress has naturally occurring anti-aging compounds that keep your skin smooth and plump. It contains important vitamins such as A, B1, B2, B6, C, E, and K that when added to diet regularly, increase the body immune system leaving the skin young and fresh.

Add the watercress to your salad topping or any other food.

- **Spinach**

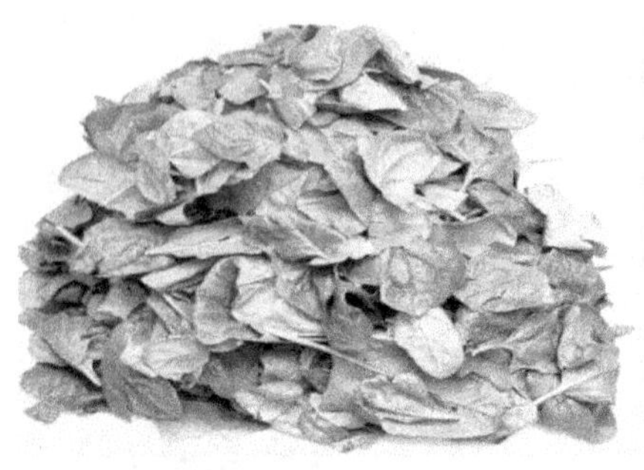

Spinach is loaded with phytonutrients that help protect the skin from damage caused by the sun. It is also rich in beta-carotene and lutein; these antioxidants help to keep the hair hydrated and improve skin elasticity. For younger skin and renewal of aging skin, add spinach to your meal regularly.

- **Red Cabbage**

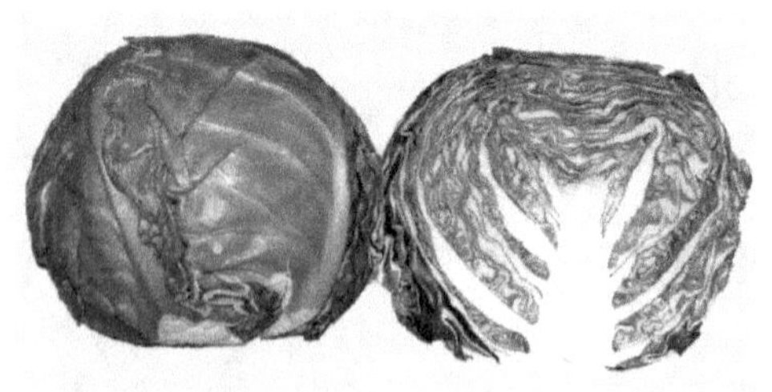

Red cabbage contains antioxidants, beta-carotene and lutein properties. These properties have an anti-aging effect on the body and also keep the body healthy.

Add red cabbage in your salad, or your daily diet to get that youthful body you so much desire.

- Cucumber

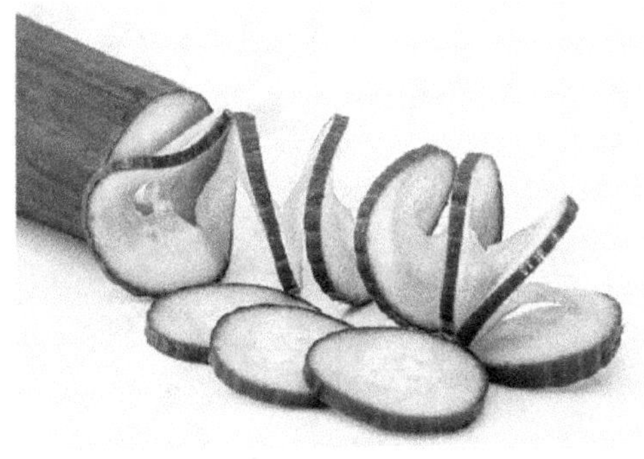

Cucumber provides the highest water content of 96% when compared to any food and water is a very important compound for anti-aging. Cucumber also contains flavonoid and tannins that prevent the harmful free radicals from entering the skin. Cucumber peels have a role to play too, and it is rich in silica, which helps the body to produce collagen that fights fine lines and wrinkles. Add slices of cucumber in your meal to enjoy the benefits.

- **Brussel Sprouts**

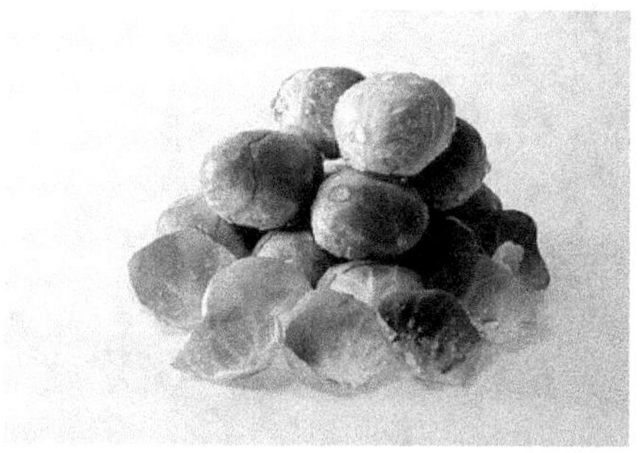

Brussel Sprouts are highly rich in vitamins C, and K. Vitamin C is an antioxidant that plays a big role in boosting the body immune system and keeping the skin healthy. Vitamin K takes care of the strength of the bone. Brussel sprouts also help in reducing oxidative stress in the cells of the skin cells.

Regular intake of brussel sprout in your diet gives your body the youthful look and strength.

- **Brinjal**

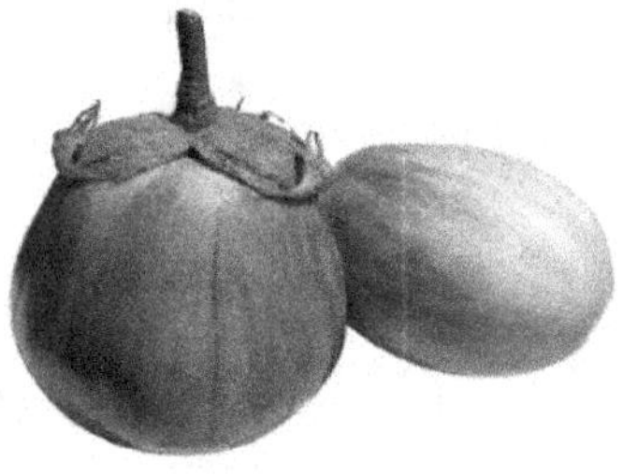

Brinjal/eggplant/aubergine is a purple vegetable high in anthocyanins. Anthocyanins are flavonoids that remove harmful free radicals from the skin, thereby keeping your skin fresh and youthful.

- **Kiwi**

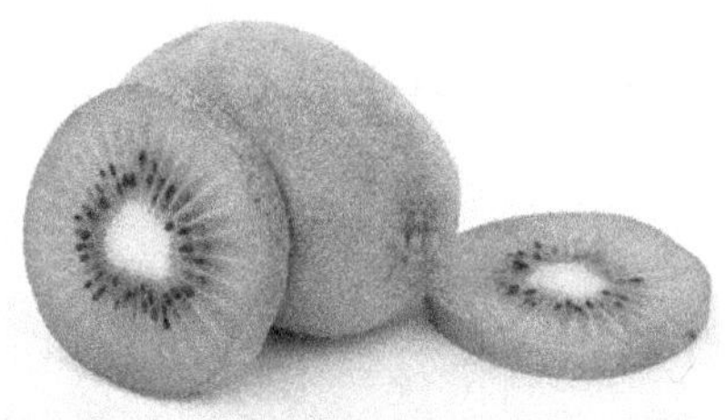

Kiwi is fully packed with many nutrients and antioxidants such as vitamin C, Vitamin E, Vitamin K, potassium, folate and fiber. These nutrients help the body to reduce the aging process. Add kiwi to your regular diet to feel young and fresh.

- **Kale**

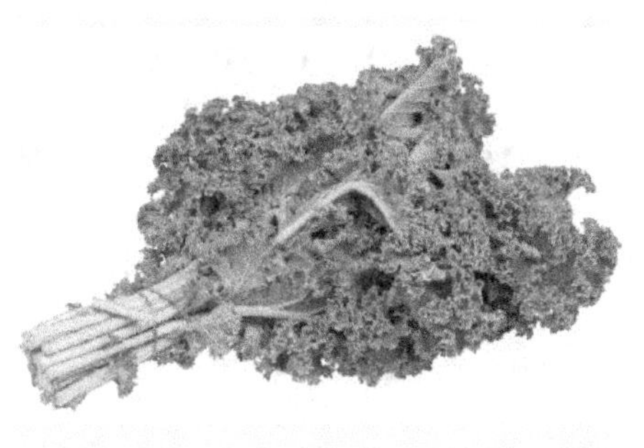

Kale is one of the ant-aging vegetables. Kale is high in all varieties of powerful anti-aging nutrients. Add it to your meal to enjoy the benefits.

- **Beets**

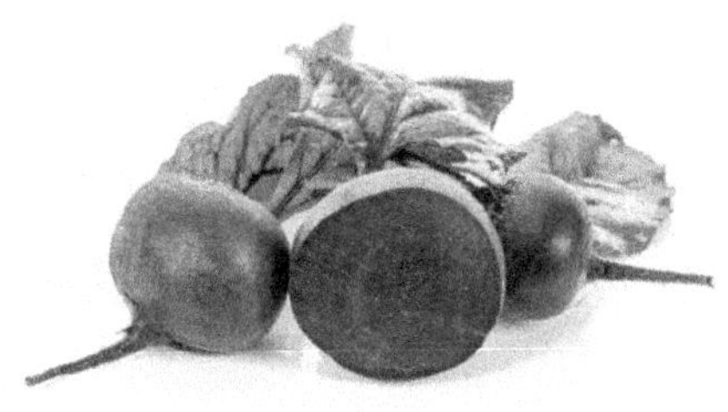

Don't let a day go without a meal of beet. Beet dilates and improves the blood flow in all area of the body, giving you that youthful look. It also contains phytonutrients that eliminate toxins from the body. Add beet to your meal daily to beat the aging effect.

Chapter Five

Herbs and Spices

- **Turmeric**

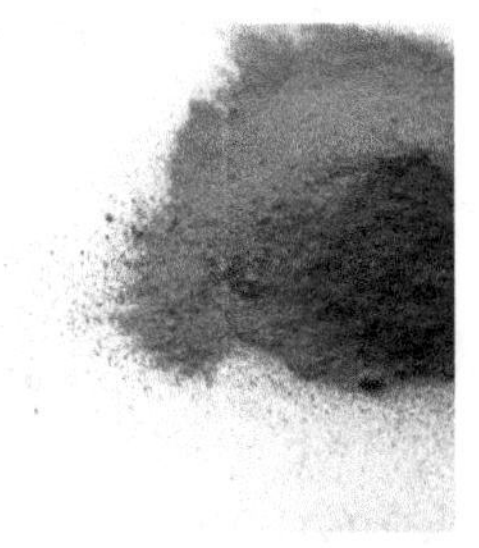

Turmeric is a potent and medicinal spice that has anti-aging properties. Turmeric contains curcumin that helps fight cell damage, chronic disease, and slowing down oxidative damage, which contributes to aging. It keeps skin and all organ aglow and in good shape. Next time you want to eat, add a pinch of turmeric in your meal for healthy cells.

- **Parsley**

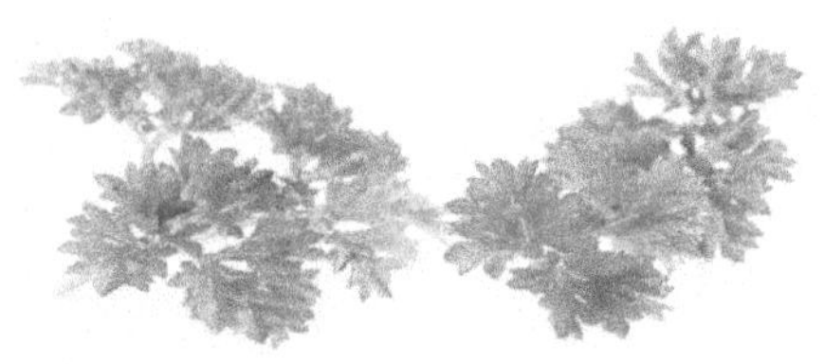

Parsley is rich in anti-oxidation property know as flavonoids. This property prevents oxidative cell damage by keeping the skin healthy and glowing. Parsley is also loaded with vitamins A, C, K, B1, and B3. Add parsley in your meal of salad bowl, smoothie, or pasta.

- **Garlic**

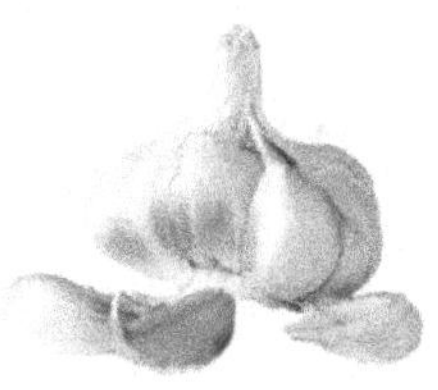

Garlic is a great spice enriched with antioxidant, detoxification and antibacterial properties that have anti-aging effects on the skin

Garlic is best when consumed raw by chopping it into smaller pieces and swallowing with water or drink.

- **Saffron**

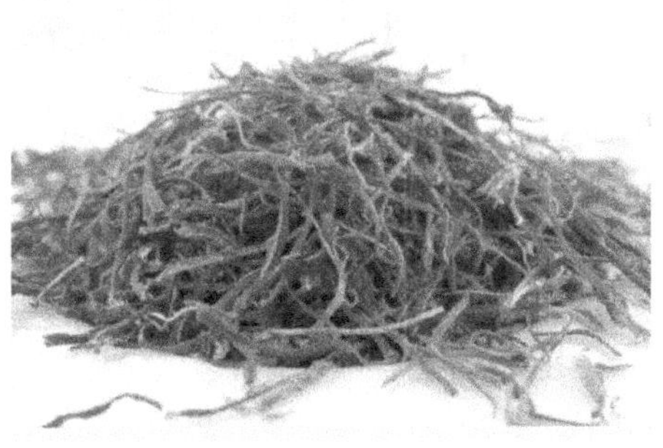

Saffron contains monoterpenoids, quercetin, and kaemferol, phenolic compounds that inhibit a process through which melanin is formed. Saffron has an anti-aging effect on the body. It also contains crocin and crocetin, a carotenoid phytonutrient with an anti-tumor and antioxidant effect, and has been proven to reduce excessive eating.

Regular consumption of saffron puts you on your toes. You can enjoy saffron by soaking a few pieces in milk and drink

- **Cilantro**

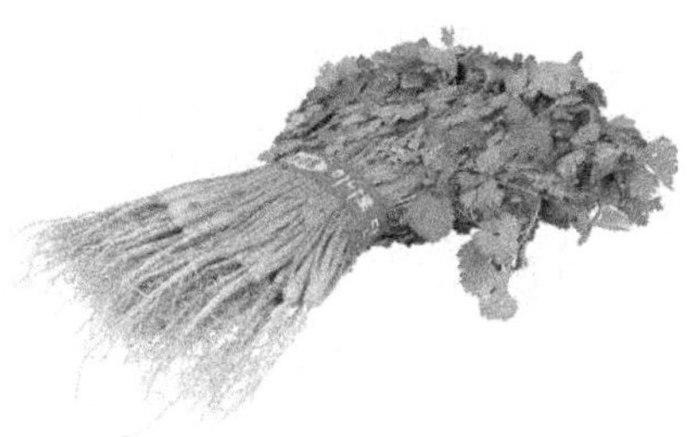

Cilantro is a green herb that contains a wide range of active phytochemicals. The phytochemicals help reduce the risk of cardiovascular disease and cancer by subduing tumor growth and cholesterol synthesis. It also supports body purifying by removing metal accumulation from the body.

- **Red bell pepper**

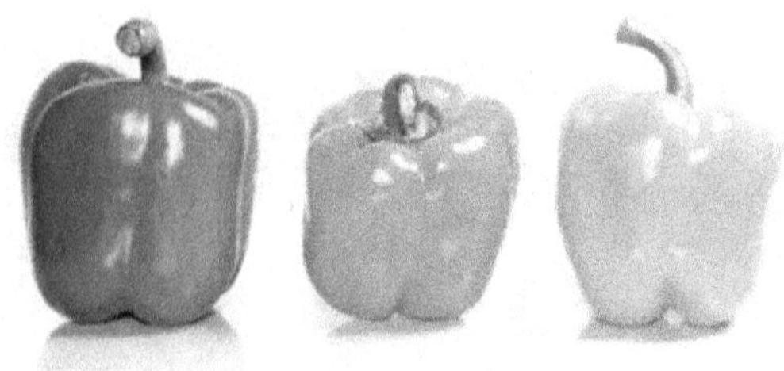

Red bell pepper has abundant of vitamin C and carotenoids. Carotenoid is an anti-inflammatory property that helps the skin to protect itself against sun damage, pollution and environmental toxins. Red, green and yellow bell peppers are the same, and each contains the same quality of wrinkle-fighting vitamin.

- **Cloves**

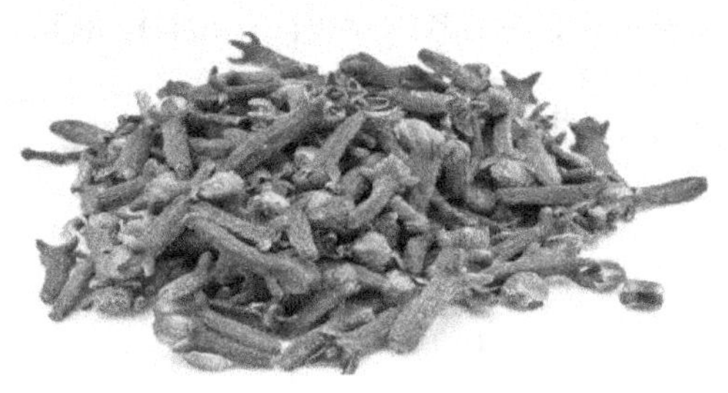

Clove is a rare spice that contains antioxidant. It helps the body to feel and look young and also shield the body from a disease such as cancer.

To consume clove, drink as a tea by allowing it to simmer in hot water for 7-10 minutes.

- **Hot Peppers**

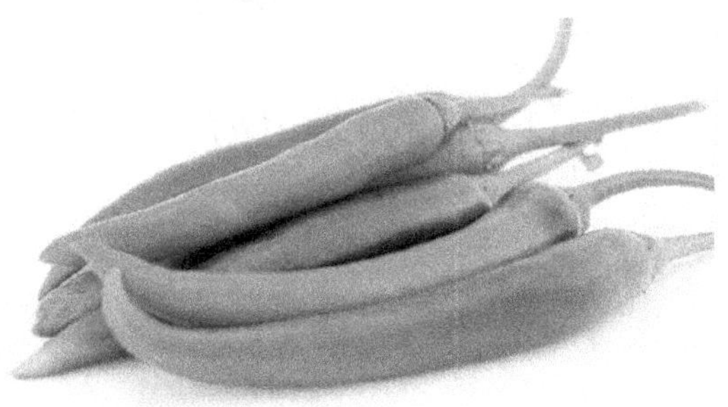

Hot pepper contains capsaicin, an antioxidant that boosts metabolism and assists your body to lose unnecessary weight. It can also improve the flow of blood in the system, keeping the body healthy and youthful. Add hot pepper as a spice in your meal and watch how it will protect you from harmful bacteria.

- **Onions**

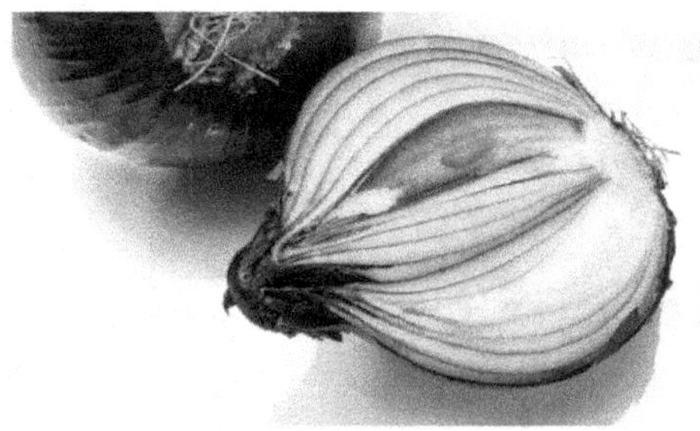

Don't let a day go by without adding onion in your meal. Onions are packed with many beneficial vitamins and minerals such as Vitamin B, Vitamin C,

Potassium, antioxidants, and other compounds. The nutrients in onions boost the body's immune system, decrease triglycerides, fight inflammation, and are outstanding for your skin and heart. Onions are great anti-aging spices that, when consumed regularly, will keep your body healthy and youthful.

Chapter Six

Oil and Honey

- **Clarified Butter (Ghee)**

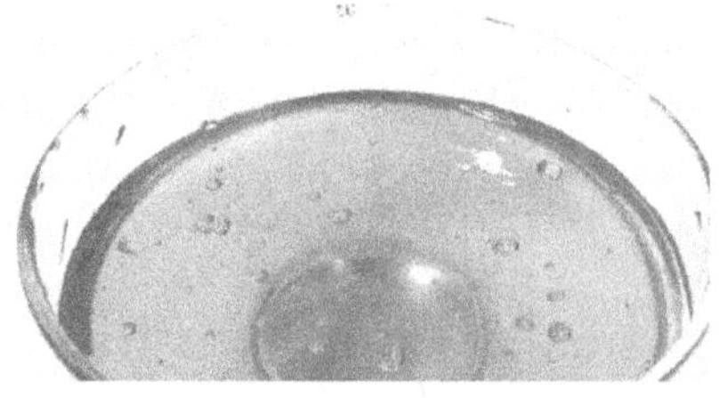

Ghee is a form of clarified butter loaded with vitamins A, C, D, E, and K. The alpha-tocopherol compound in ghee protects the skin from damage and keeps it young. Ghee is made from high-quality organic butter that contains a lot of healthy fat that work to keep your skin smooth and soft.

- **Manuka honey**

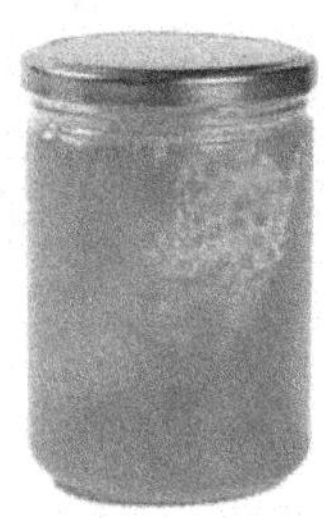

Manuka honey is a known name in natural skin products. It boosts cytokine production, which works is to fight off pathogens and protects the body from infections. It is also a natural remedy for boosting the immune system and rejuvenating skin from harmful pollutants in the air. Add manuka honey in your next cup of tea and enjoy the benefits.

- **Olive Oil**

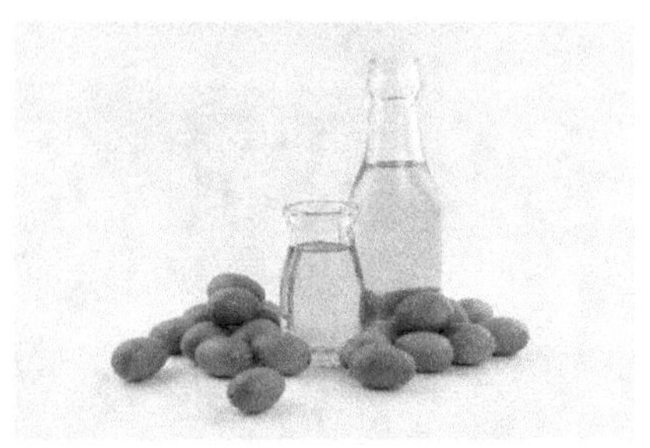

Extra virgin olive oil contains a high amount of oleic acid, which slows the effect of C-reactive protein, playing a vital role in age-related issues. It weakens the process of cell regeneration in the body, thereby keeping your skin youthful and healthy.

Add extra virgin oil to your meal instead of butter or mayo anytime you want to cook and experience an anti-aging effect.

Chapter Seven

Beverages

- **Green Tea**

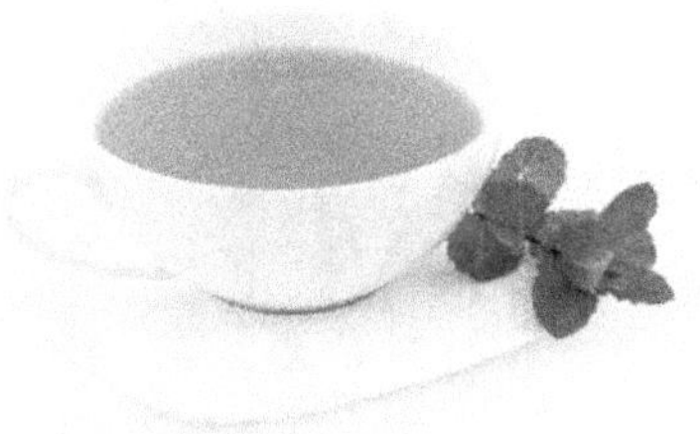

Green tea is packed with a powerful antioxidant like polyphenols and flavonoids. Polyphenols increase the production of keratinocytes by slowing down the effect of aging on the skin. At the same time, flavonoids protect the body against diseases and block harmful free radicals that damage the body. For a wrinkle-free and youthful look, make sure you drink at least on teacup of green tea every day in the early morning.

- **Red Wine**

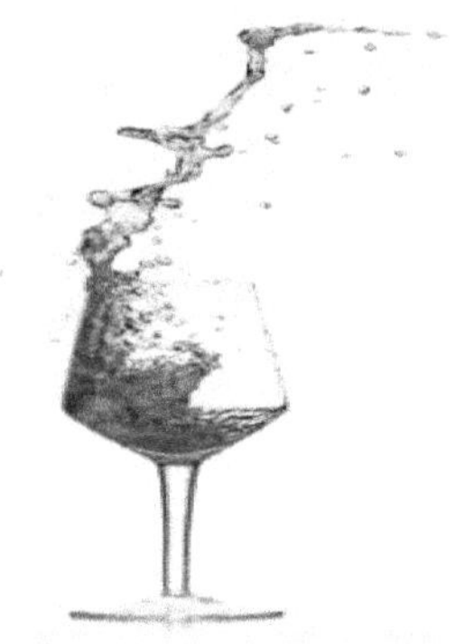

Yes, red wine is not left out. It contains a powerful anti-aging oxidant known as resveratrol, which is good for the brain, heart, muscle, and other part of the body. Red wine also contains flavonoids, which reduces bad cholesterol to boost good cholesterol. It rejuvenates the cells and reduces the effect of aging on the skin.

It times to start pouring and drinking in moderation to avoid the negative effect that comes with over-drinking.

- **Almond Milk**

Almond milk contains a high amount of vitamin E, and it is suitable for those who dislike dairy or want to avoid it. It rejuvenates the skin and gives you that youthful look.

- **Greek yogurt**

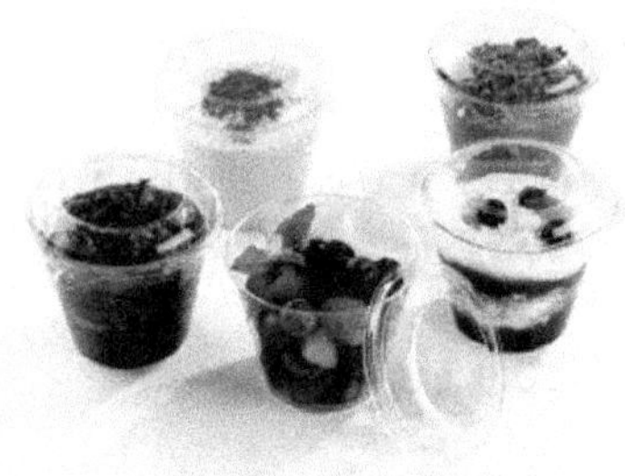

Yogurt is a low-fat snack packed with protein, vitamin C, and D. These vitamins are essential for maintaining healthy bones as you grow older and particularly after menopause.

Yogurt is great for keeping cells young and skin glowing because it contains gut-friendly bacteria that behave as probiotics. The work of probiotics is to slow down both inner and outer aging.

You can eat unsweetened or plain yogurt
and add a bit of blueberry or your
favorites fruit.

Chapter Eight

Sea foods

- **Salmon**

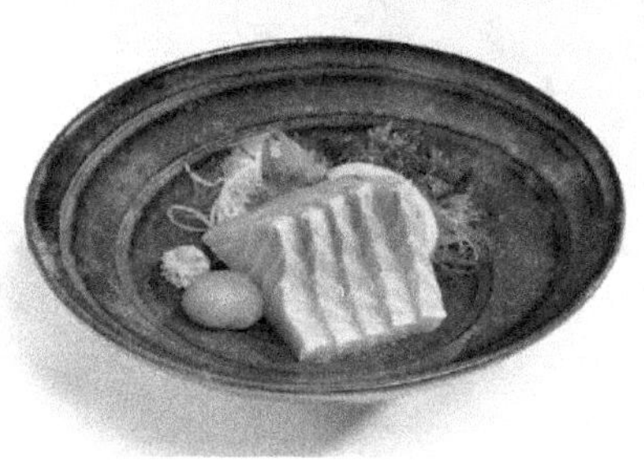

Salmon and other cold-water fish (sardines and mackerel) are enriched with Astaxanthin, a compound that prevents inflammation and decreases oxidative stress by slowing down the effects of aging. Salmon is also enriched with omega-3 fatty acid and selenium. Regular addition of these foods in your meal help strengthens weakening membranes thereby, reducing redness and inflammation. You can have salmon grilled or baked or broil it with spices and butter.

- **Oysters**

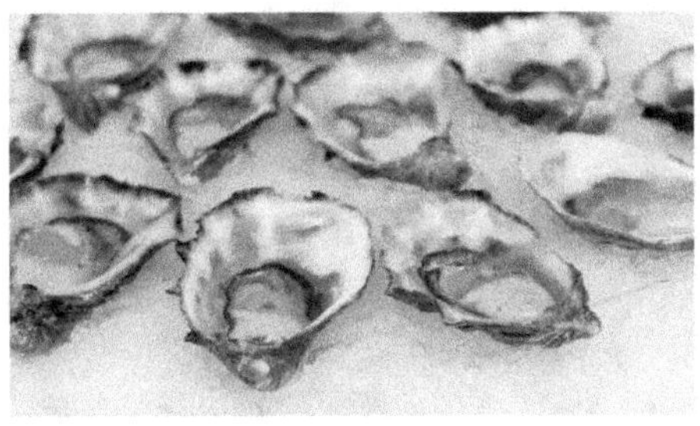

Oysters are one of the shellfish that are high in copper and zinc. These minerals help prevent the early onset of wrinkles, ward off osteoporosis and joint pain, balance hormones, and prevent diseases. It gives the body youthful skin.

Next time you visit that restaurant, request for a plate of an oyster.

Chapter Nine

Others

- **Maca**

Maca root contains polyphenol antioxidants that, when applied to the skin, prevent skin from damage caused by UV rays exposure. Maca is an anti-aging superfood with tremendous health benefits. It is loaded with energy-giving nutrients, boost libido, and improves mood.

Add a teaspoon of maca powder to your morning coffee and enjoy the benefits.

- **Dark chocolate**

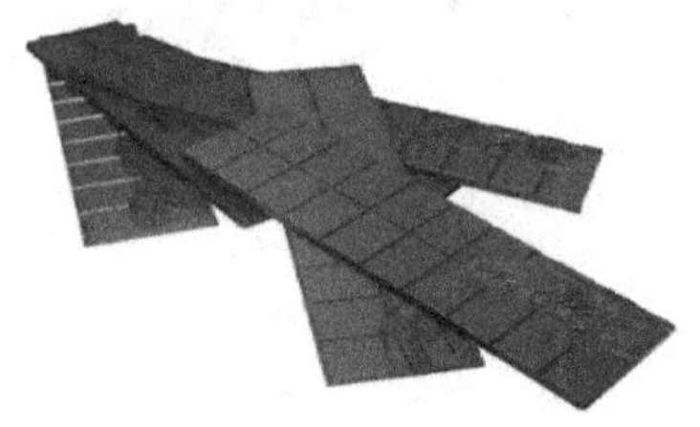

Dark chocolate contains many flavonols, and its regular intake prevents an increase in wrinkles and maintains hydration levels and skin elasticity, especially in the anti-aging realm. The flavonols present in dark chocolate are beneficial to the body's appearance by increasing the rate of blood flow to the skin.

It also prevents the damage that is caused by UV radiation.

Eat dark chocolate or use it to garnish morning bowl of oatmeal, cereals and cakes.

- **Sweet potatoes**

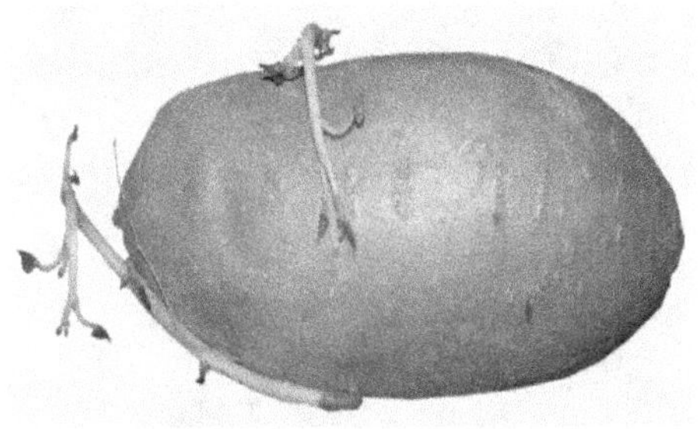

This tasty variety of potato is loaded with vitamin A. Vitamin A nutrient helps to revitalize damaged collagen in the skin by ultimately fighting off fine lines and wrinkles, and it also brightens skin's complexion. Regular consumption of cooked or baked potato reduces the effect of aging.

- **Lean beef**

Beef is high in protein, which works to maintain the collagen that keeps the body healthy and the skin youthful. Eating a little serving of meat per week can alter the negative effects of aging on your skin.

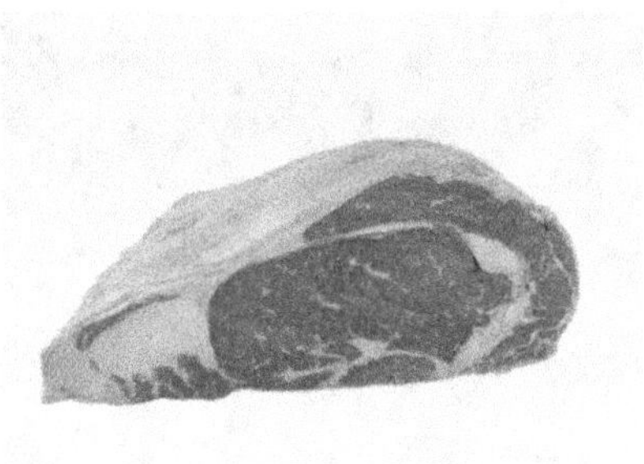